What is autism spectrum dis

Autism is a group of developmental brain disorders, collec
(ASD). The term "spectrum" refers to the wide range of symptoms, skills, and levels of impairment, or disability, that children with ASD can have. Some children are mildly impaired by their symptoms, but others are severely disabled.

ASD is diagnosed according to guidelines listed in the *Diagnostic and Statistical Manual of Mental Disorders, Fourth Edition - Text Revision* (DSM-IV-TR).[1] The manual currently defines five disorders, sometimes called pervasive developmental disorders (PDDs), as ASD:

- Autistic disorder (classic autism)
- Asperger's disorder (Asperger syndrome)
- Pervasive developmental disorder not otherwise specified (PDD-NOS)
- Rett's disorder (Rett syndrome)
- Childhood disintegrative disorder (CDD).

This information packet will focus on autism, Asperger syndrome, and PDD-NOS, with brief descriptions of Rett syndrome and CDD in the section, "Related disorders." Information can also be found on the *Eunice Kennedy Shriver* National Institute of Child Health and Human Development website at http://www.nichd.nih.gov and the Centers for Disease Control and Prevention website at http://www.cdc.gov/ncbddd/autism/index.html.

What are the symptoms of ASD?

Symptoms of autism spectrum disorder (ASD) vary from one child to the next, but in general, they fall into three areas:

- Social impairment
- Communication difficulties
- Repetitive and stereotyped behaviors.

Children with ASD do not follow typical patterns when developing social and communication skills. Parents are usually the first to notice unusual behaviors in their child. Often, certain behaviors become more noticeable when comparing children of the same age.

In some cases, babies with ASD may seem different very early in their development. Even before their first birthday, some babies become overly focused on certain objects, rarely make eye contact, and fail to engage in typical back-and-forth play and babbling with their parents. Other children may develop normally until the second or even third year of life, but then start to lose interest in others and become silent, withdrawn, or indifferent to social signals. Loss or reversal of normal development is called regression and occurs in some children with ASD.[2]

Social impairment

Most children with ASD have trouble engaging in everyday social interactions. According to the *Diagnostic and Statistical Manual of Mental Disorders, Fourth Edition - Text Revision*, some children with ASD may:

- Make little eye contact
- Tend to look and listen less to people in their environment or fail to respond to other people
- Do not readily seek to share their enjoyment of toys or activities by pointing or showing things to others
- Respond unusually when others show anger, distress, or affection.

Recent research suggests that children with ASD do not respond to emotional cues in human social interactions because they may not pay attention to the social cues that others typically notice. For example, one study found that children with ASD focus on the mouth of the person speaking to them instead of on the eyes (article at http://www.nimh.nih.gov/science-news/2008/lack-of-eye-contact-may-predict-level-of-social-disability-in-two-year-olds-with-autism.shtml), which is where children with typical development tend to focus.[3] A related study showed that children with ASD appear to be drawn to repetitive movements linked to a sound, such as hand-clapping during a game of pat-a-cake (article at http://www.nimh.nih.gov/science-news/2009/autism-skews-developing-brain-with-synchronous-motion-and-sound.shtml).[4] More research is needed to confirm these findings, but such studies suggest that children with ASD may misread or not notice subtle social cues—a smile, a wink, or a grimace—that could help them understand social relationships and interactions. For these children, a question such as, "Can you wait a minute?" always means the same thing, whether the speaker is joking, asking a real question, or issuing a firm request. Without the ability to interpret another person's tone of voice as well as gestures, facial expressions, and other nonverbal communications, children with ASD may not properly respond.

Likewise, it can be hard for others to understand the body language of children with ASD. Their facial expressions, movements, and gestures are often vague or do not match what they are saying. Their tone of voice may not reflect their actual feelings either. Many older children with ASD speak with an unusual tone of voice and may sound sing-song or flat and robotlike.[1]

Children with ASD also may have trouble understanding another person's point of view. For example, by school age, most children understand that other people have different information, feelings, and goals than they have. Children with ASD may lack this understanding, leaving them unable to predict or understand other people's actions.

Communication issues

According to the American Academy of Pediatrics' developmental milestones, by the first birthday, typical toddlers can say one or two words, turn when they hear their name, and point when they want a toy. When offered something they do not want, toddlers make it clear with words, gestures, or facial expressions that the answer is "no."

For children with ASD, reaching such milestones may not be so straightforward. For example, some children with autism may:

- Fail or be slow to respond to their name or other verbal attempts to gain their attention
- Fail or be slow to develop gestures, such as pointing and showing things to others

- Coo and babble in the first year of life, but then stop doing so
- Develop language at a delayed pace
- Learn to communicate using pictures or their own sign language
- Speak only in single words or repeat certain phrases over and over, seeming unable to combine words into meaningful sentences
- Repeat words or phrases that they hear, a condition called echolalia
- Use words that seem odd, out of place, or have a special meaning known only to those familiar with the child's way of communicating.

Even children with ASD who have relatively good language skills often have difficulties with the back and forth of conversations. For example, because they find it difficult to understand and react to social cues, children with Asperger syndrome often talk at length about a favorite subject, but they won't allow anyone else a chance to respond or notice when others react indifferently.[1]

Children with ASD who have not yet developed meaningful gestures or language may simply scream or grab or otherwise act out until they are taught better ways to express their needs. As these children grow up, they can become aware of their difficulty in understanding others and in being understood. This awareness may cause them to become anxious or depressed. For more information on mental health issues in children with ASD, see the section: What are some other conditions that children with ASD may have?

Repetitive and stereotyped behaviors

Children with ASD often have repetitive motions or unusual behaviors. These behaviors may be extreme and very noticeable, or they can be mild and discreet. For example, some children may repeatedly flap their arms or walk in specific patterns, while others may subtly move their fingers by their eyes in what looks to be a gesture. These repetitive actions are sometimes called "stereotypy" or "stereotyped behaviors."

Children with ASD also tend to have overly focused interests. Children with ASD may become fascinated with moving objects or parts of objects, like the wheels on a moving car. They might spend a long time lining up toys in a certain way, rather than playing with them. They may also become very upset if someone accidentally moves one of the toys. Repetitive behavior can also take the form of a persistent, intense preoccupation.[1] For example, they might be obsessed with learning all about vacuum cleaners, train schedules, or lighthouses. Children with ASD often have great interest in numbers, symbols, or science topics.

While children with ASD often do best with routine in their daily activities and surroundings, inflexibility may often be extreme and cause serious difficulties. They may insist on eating the same exact meals every day or taking the same exact route to school. A slight change in a specific routine can be extremely upsetting.[1] Some children may even have emotional outbursts, especially when feeling angry or frustrated or when placed in a new or stimulating environment.

No two children express exactly the same types and severity of symptoms. In fact, many typically developing children occasionally display some of the behaviors common to children with ASD. However, if you notice your child has several ASD-related symptoms, have your child screened and evaluated by a health professional experienced with ASD.

Related disorders

Rett syndrome and childhood disintegrative disorder (CDD) are two very rare forms of ASD that include a regression in development. Only 1 of every 10,000 to 22,000 girls has Rett syndrome.[5,6] Even rarer, only 1 or 2 out of 100,000 children with ASD have CDD.[7]

Unlike other forms of ASD, Rett syndrome mostly affects girls. In general, children with Rett syndrome develop normally for 6–18 months before regression and autism-like symptoms begin to appear. Children with Rett syndrome may also have difficulties with coordination, movement, and speech. Physical, occupational, and speech therapy can help, but no specific treatment for Rett syndrome is available yet.

With funding from the *Eunice Kennedy Shriver* National Institute of Child Health and Human Development, scientists have discovered that a mutation in the sequence of a single gene is linked to most cases of Rett syndrome.[8] This discovery may help scientists find ways to slow or stop the progress of the disorder. It may also improve doctors' ability to diagnose and treat children with Rett syndrome earlier, improving their overall quality of life.

CDD affects very few children, which makes it hard for researchers to learn about the disease. Symptoms of CDD may appear by age 2, but the average age of onset is between age 3 and 4. Until this time, children with CDD usually have age-appropriate communication and social skills. The long period of normal development before regression helps to set CDD apart from Rett syndrome. CDD may affect boys more often than girls.[9]

Children with CDD experience severe, wide-ranging and obvious loss of previously-obtained motor, language, and social skills.[10] The loss of such skills as vocabulary is more dramatic in CDD than in classic autism.[11] Other symptoms of CDD include loss of bowel and bladder control.[1]

How is ASD diagnosed?

ASD diagnosis is often a two-stage process. The first stage involves general developmental screening during well-child checkups with a pediatrician or an early childhood health care provider. Children who show some developmental problems are referred for additional evaluation. The second stage involves a thorough evaluation by a team of doctors and other health professionals with a wide range of specialities.[12] At this stage, a child may be diagnosed as having autism or another developmental disorder.

Children with autism spectrum disorder (ASD) can usually be reliably diagnosed by age 2, though research suggests that some screening tests can be helpful at 18 months or even younger.[12, 13]

Many people—including pediatricians, family doctors, teachers, and parents—may minimize signs of ASD at first, believing that children will "catch up" with their peers. While you may be concerned about labeling your young child with ASD, the earlier the disorder is diagnosed, the sooner specific interventions may begin. Early intervention can reduce or prevent the more severe disabilities associated with ASD. Early intervention may also improve your child's IQ, language, and everyday functional skills, also called adaptive behavior.[14]

Screening

A well-child checkup should include a developmental screening test, with specific ASD screening at 18 and 24 months as recommended by the American Academy of Pediatrics.[14] Screening for ASD is not the same as diagnosing ASD. Screening instruments are used as a first step to

Types of ASD screening instruments

Sometimes the doctor will ask parents questions about the child's symptoms to screen for ASD. Other screening instruments combine information from parents with the doctor's own observations of the child. Examples of screening instruments for toddlers and preschoolers include:

- Checklist of Autism in Toddlers (CHAT)
- Modified Checklist for Autism in Toddlers (M-CHAT)
- Screening Tool for Autism in Two-Year-Olds (STAT)
- Social Communication Questionnaire (SCQ)
- Communication and Symbolic Behavior Scales (CSBS).

To screen for mild ASD or Asperger syndrome in older children, the doctor may rely on different screening instruments, such as:

- Autism Spectrum Screening Questionnaire (ASSQ)
- Australian Scale for Asperger's Syndrome (ASAS)
- Childhood Asperger Syndrome Test (CAST).

Some helpful resources on ASD screening include the Center for Disease Control and Prevention's General Developmental Screening tools and ASD Specific Screening tools on their website at http://cdc.gov/ncbddd/autism/screening.html.

tell the doctor whether a child needs more testing. If your child's pediatrician does not routinely screen your child for ASD, ask that it be done.

For parents, your own experiences and concerns about your child's development will be very important in the screening process. Keep your own notes about your child's development and look through family videos, photos, and baby albums to help you remember when you first noticed each behavior and when your child reached certain developmental milestones.

Comprehensive diagnostic evaluation

The second stage of diagnosis must be thorough in order to find whether other conditions may be causing your child's symptoms. For more information, see the section: What are some other conditions that children with ASD may have?

A team that includes a psychologist, a neurologist, a psychiatrist, a speech therapist, or other professionals experienced in diagnosing ASD may do this evaluation. The evaluation may assess the child's cognitive level (thinking skills), language level, and adaptive behavior (age-appropriate skills needed to complete daily activities independently, for example eating, dressing, and toileting).

Because ASD is a complex disorder that sometimes occurs along with other illnesses or learning disorders, the comprehensive evaluation may include brain imaging and gene tests, along with in-depth memory, problem-solving, and language testing.[12] Children with any delayed development should also get a hearing test and be screened for lead poisoning as part of the comprehensive evaluation.

Although children can lose their hearing along with developing ASD, common ASD symptoms (such as not turning to face a person calling their name) can also make it seem that children cannot hear when in fact they can. If a child is not responding to speech, especially to his or her name, it's important for the doctor to test whether a child has hearing loss.

The evaluation process is a good time for parents and caregivers to ask questions and get advice from the whole evaluation team. The outcome of the evaluation will help plan for treatment and interventions to help your child. Be sure to ask who you can contact with follow-up questions.

What are some other conditions that children with ASD may have?

Sensory problems

Many children with autism spectrum disorder (ASD) either overreact or underreact to certain sights, sounds, smells, textures, and tastes. For example, some may:

- Dislike or show discomfort from a light touch or the feel of clothes on their skin
- Experience pain from certain sounds, like a vacuum cleaner, a ringing telephone, or a sudden storm; sometimes they will cover their ears and scream
- Have no reaction to intense cold or pain.

Researchers are trying to determine if these unusual reactions are related to differences in integrating multiple types of information from the senses.

Sleep problems

Children with ASD tend to have problems falling asleep or staying asleep, or have other sleep problems.[15] These problems make it harder for them to pay attention, reduce their ability to function, and lead to poor behavior. In addition, parents of children with ASD and sleep problems tend to report greater family stress and poorer overall health among themselves.

Fortunately, sleep problems can often be treated with changes in behavior, such as following a sleep schedule or creating a bedtime routine. Some children may sleep better using medications such as melatonin, which is a hormone that helps regulate the body's sleep-wake cycle. Like any medication, melatonin can have unwanted side effects. Talk to your child's doctor about possible risks and benefits before giving your child melatonin. Treating sleep problems in children with ASD may improve the child's overall behavior and functioning, as well as relieve family stress.[16]

Intellectual disability

Many children with ASD have some degree of intellectual disability. When tested, some areas of ability may be normal, while others—especially cognitive (thinking) and language abilities—may be relatively weak. For example, a child with ASD may do well on tasks related to sight (such as putting a puzzle together) but may not do as well on language-based problem-solving tasks. Children with a form of ASD like Asperger syndrome often have average or above-average language skills and do not show delays in cognitive ability or speech.

Seizures

One in four children with ASD has seizures, often starting either in early childhood or during the teen years.[17] Seizures, caused by abnormal electrical activity in the brain, can result in

- A short-term loss of consciousness, or a blackout
- Convulsions, which are uncontrollable shaking of the whole body, or unusual movements
- Staring spells.

Sometimes lack of sleep or a high fever can trigger a seizure. An electroencephalogram (EEG), a nonsurgical test that records electrical activity in the brain, can help confirm whether a child is having seizures. However, some children with ASD have abnormal EEGs even if they are not having seizures.

Seizures can be treated with medicines called anticonvulsants. Some seizure medicines affect behavior; changes in behavior should be closely watched in children with ASD. In most cases, a doctor will use the lowest dose of medicine that works for the child. Anticonvulsants usually reduce the number of seizures but may not prevent all of them.

For more information about medications, see the NIMH online booklet, "Medications" at http://www.nimh.nih.gov/health/publications/mental-health-medications/index.shtml. None of these medications have been approved by the FDA to specifically treat symptoms of ASD.

Fragile X syndrome

Fragile X syndrome is a genetic disorder and is the most common form of inherited intellectual disability,[18] causing symptoms similar to ASD. The name refers to one part of the X chromosome that has a defective piece that appears pinched and fragile when viewed with a microscope. Fragile X syndrome results from a change, called a mutation, on a single gene. This mutation, in effect, turns off the gene. Some people may have only a small mutation and not show any symptoms, while others have a larger mutation and more severe symptoms.[19]

Around 1 in 3 children who have Fragile X syndrome also meet the diagnostic criteria for ASD, and about 1 in 25 children diagnosed with ASD have the mutation that causes Fragile X syndrome.[19]

Because this disorder is inherited, children with ASD should be checked for Fragile X, especially if the parents want to have more children. Other family members who are planning to have children may also want to be checked for Fragile X syndrome. For more information on Fragile X, see the *Eunice Kennedy Shriver* National Institute of Child Health and Human Development website at http://www.nichd.nih.gov/health/topics/fragile_x_syndrome.cfm.

Tuberous sclerosis

Tuberous sclerosis is a rare genetic disorder that causes noncancerous tumors to grow in the brain and other vital organs. Tuberous sclerosis occurs in 1 to 4 percent of people with ASD.[18, 20] A genetic mutation causes the disorder, which has also been linked to mental retardation, epilepsy, and many other physical and mental health problems. There is no cure for tuberous sclerosis, but many symptoms can be treated.

Gastrointestinal problems

Some parents of children with ASD report that their child has frequent gastrointestinal (GI) or digestion problems, including stomach pain, diarrhea, constipation, acid reflux, vomiting, or bloating. Food allergies may also cause problems for children with ASD.[21] It's unclear whether children with ASD are more likely to have GI problems than typically developing children.[22, 23] If your child has GI problems, a doctor who specializes in GI problems, called a gastroenterologist, can help find the cause and suggest appropriate treatment.

Some studies have reported that children with ASD seem to have more GI symptoms, but these findings may not apply to all children with ASD. For example, a recent study found that children with ASD in Minnesota were more likely to have physical and behavioral difficulties related to diet (for example, lactose intolerance or insisting on certain foods), as well as constipation, than children without ASD.[23] The researchers suggested that children with ASD may not have underlying GI problems, but that their behavior may create GI symptoms—for example, a child who insists on eating only certain foods may not get enough fiber or fluids in his or her diet, which leads to constipation.

Some parents may try to put their child on a special diet to control ASD or GI symptoms. While some children may benefit from limiting certain foods, there is no strong evidence that these special diets reduce ASD symptoms.[24] If you want to try a special diet, first talk with a doctor or a nutrition expert to make sure your child's nutritional needs are being met.

Co-occurring mental disorders

Children with ASD can also develop mental disorders such as anxiety disorders, attention deficit hyperactivity disorder (ADHD), or depression. Research shows that people with ASD are at higher risk for some mental disorders than people without ASD.[25] Managing these co-occurring conditions with medications or behavioral therapy, which teaches children how to control their behavior, can reduce symptoms that appear to worsen a child's ASD symptoms. Controlling these conditions will allow children with ASD to focus more on managing the ASD.[26]

How is ASD treated?

While there's no proven cure yet for autism spectrum disorder (ASD), treating ASD early, using school-based programs, and getting proper medical care can greatly reduce ASD symptoms and increase your child's ability to grow and learn new skills.

Early intervention

Research has shown that intensive behavioral therapy during the toddler or preschool years can significantly improve cognitive and language skills in young children with ASD.[27, 28] There is no single best treatment for all children with ASD, but the American Academy of Pediatrics recently noted common features of effective early intervention programs.[29] These include:

- Starting as soon as a child has been diagnosed with ASD
- Providing focused and challenging learning activities at the proper developmental level for the child for at least 25 hours per week and 12 months per year
- Having small classes to allow each child to have one-on-one time with the therapist or teacher and small group learning activities
- Having special training for parents and family
- Encouraging activities that include typically developing children, as long as such activities help meet a specific learning goal
- Measuring and recording each child's progress and adjusting the intervention program as needed
- Providing a high degree of structure, routine, and visual cues, such as posted activity schedules and clearly defined boundaries, to reduce distractions
- Guiding the child in adapting learned skills to new situations and settings and maintaining learned skills
- Using a curriculum that focuses on
  - Language and communication
  - Social skills, such as joint attention (looking at other people to draw attention to something interesting and share in experiencing it)
  - Self-help and daily living skills, such as dressing and grooming
  - Research-based methods to reduce challenging behaviors, such as aggression and tantrums
  - Cognitive skills, such as pretend play or seeing someone else's point of view
  - Typical school-readiness skills, such as letter recognition and counting.

One type of a widely accepted treatment is applied behavior analysis (ABA). The goals of ABA are to shape and reinforce new behaviors, such as learning to speak and play, and reduce undesirable ones. ABA, which can involve intensive, one-on-one child-teacher interaction for up to 40 hours a week, has inspired the development of other, similar interventions that aim to help those with ASD reach their full potential.[30, 31] ABA-based interventions include:

- **Verbal Behavior**—focuses on teaching language using a sequenced curriculum that guides children from simple verbal behaviors (echoing) to more functional communication skills through techniques such as errorless teaching and prompting[32]

- **Pivotal Response Training**—aims at identifying pivotal skills, such as initiation and self-management, that affect a broad range of behavioral responses. This intervention incorporates parent and family education aimed at providing skills that enable the child to function in inclusive settings.[33, 34]

Other types of early interventions include:

- **Developmental, Individual Difference, Relationship-based(DIR)/ Floortime Model**—aims to build healthy and meaningful relationships and abilities by following the natural emotions and interests of the child.[35] One particular example is the Early Start Denver Model, which fosters improvements in communication, thinking, language, and other social skills and seeks to reduce atypical behaviors. Using developmental and relationship-based approaches, this therapy can be delivered in natural settings such as the home or pre-school.[33, 34]

- **TEACCH (Treatment and Education of Autistic and related Communication handicapped Children)**—emphasizes adapting the child's physical environment and using visual cues (for example, having classroom materials clearly marked and located so that students can access them independently). Using individualized plans for each student, TEACCH builds on the child's strengths and emerging skills.[34, 36]

- **Interpersonal Synchrony**—targets social development and imitation skills, and focuses on teaching children how to establish and maintain engagement with others.

For children younger than age 3, these interventions usually take place at home or in a child care center. Because parents are a child's earliest teachers, more programs are beginning to train parents to continue the therapy at home.

Students with ASD may benefit from some type of social skills training program.[37] While these programs need more research, they generally seek to increase and improve skills necessary for creating positive social interactions and avoiding negative responses. For example, Children's Friendship Training focuses on improving children's conversation and interaction skills and teaches them how to make friends, be a good sport, and respond appropriately to teasing.[38]

Working with your child's school

Start by speaking with your child's teacher, school counselor, or the school's student support team to begin an evaluation. Each state has a Parent Training and Information Center and a Protection and Advocacy Agency that can help you get an evaluation. A team of professionals conducts the evaluation using a variety of tools and measures. The evaluation will look at all areas related to your child's abilities and needs.

Once your child has been evaluated, he or she has several options, depending on the specific needs. If your child needs special education services and is eligible under the Individuals with Disabilities Education Act (IDEA), the school district (or the government agency administering the program) must develop an individualized education plan, or IEP specifically for your child within 30 days.

IDEA provides free screenings and early intervention services to children from birth to age 3. IDEA also provides special education and related services from ages 3 to 21. Information is available from the U.S. Department of Education at http://idea.ed.gov.

If your child is not eligible for special education services—not all children with ASD are eligible—he or she can still get free public education suited to his or her needs, which is available to all public-school children with disabilities under Section 504 of the Rehabilitation Act of 1973, regardless of the type or severity of the disability.

The U.S. Department of Education's Office for Civil Rights enforces Section 504 in programs and activities that receive Federal education funds. For more information on Section 504, please see http://www.ed.gov/about/offices/list/ocr/504faq.html.

More information about U.S. Department of Education programs for children with disabilities is available at http://www.ed.gov/parents/needs/speced/edpicks.jhtml?src=ln.

During middle and high school years, your child's teachers will begin to discuss practical issues such as work, living away from a parent or caregiver's home, and hobbies. These lessons should include gaining work experience, using public transportation, and learning skills that will be important in community living.[29]

Medications

Some medications can help reduce symptoms that cause problems for your child in school or at home. Many other medications may be prescribed off-label, meaning they have not been approved by the U.S. Food and Drug Administration (FDA) for a certain use or for certain people. Doctors may prescribe medications off-label if they have been approved to treat other disorders that have similar symptoms to ASD, or if they have been effective in treating adults or older children with ASD. Doctors prescribe medications off-label to try to help the youngest patients, but more research is needed to be sure that these medicines are safe and effective for children and teens with ASD.

At this time, the only medications approved by the FDA to treat aspects of ASD are the antipsychotics risperidone (Risperdal) and aripripazole (Abilify). These medications can help reduce irritability—meaning aggression, self-harming acts, or temper tantrums—in children ages 5 to 16 who have ASD.

Some medications that may be prescribed off-label for children with ASD include the following:

- **Antipsychotic medications** are more commonly used to treat serious mental illnesses such as schizophrenia. These medicines may help reduce aggression and other serious behavioral problems in children, including children with ASD. They may also help reduce repetitive behaviors, hyperactivity, and attention problems.[29]

- **Antidepressant medications**, such as fluoxetine (Prozac) or sertraline (Zoloft), are usually prescribed to treat depression and anxiety but are sometimes prescribed to reduce repetitive behaviors. Some antidepressants may also help control aggression and anxiety in children with ASD.[29] However, researchers still are not sure if these medications are useful; a recent study suggested that the antidepressant citalopram (Celexa) was no more effective than a placebo (sugar pill) at reducing repetitive behaviors in children with ASD (see article at http://www.nimh.nih.gov/science-news/2009/citalopram-no-better-than-placebo-treatment-for-children-with-autism-spectrum-disorders.shtml).[39]

- **Stimulant medications**, such as methylphenidate (Ritalin), are safe and effective in treating people with attention deficit hyperactivity disorder (ADHD). Methylphenidate has been shown to effectively treat hyperactivity in children with ASD as well. But not as many children with ASD respond to treatment, and those who do have shown more side effects than children with ADHD and not ASD.[40]

All medications carry a risk of side effects. For details on the side effects of common psychiatric medications, see the NIMH website on "Medications" at http://www.nimh.nih.gov/health/publications/mental-health-medications/index.shtml.

FDA warning about antidepressants

Antidepressants are safe and popular, but some studies have suggested that they may have unintended effects on some people, especially in teens and young adults. The FDA warning says that patients of all ages taking antidepressants should be watched closely, especially during the first few weeks of treatment. Possible side effects to look for are depression that gets worse, suicidal thinking or behavior, or any unusual changes in behavior such as trouble sleeping, agitation, or withdrawal from normal social situations. Families and caregivers should report any changes to the doctor. The latest information from the FDA can be found at http://www.fda.gov.

A child with ASD may not respond in the same way to medications as typically developing children. You should work with a doctor who has experience treating children with ASD. The doctor will usually start your child on the lowest dose that helps control problem symptoms. Ask the doctor about any side effects of the medication and keep a record of how your child reacts to the medication. The doctor should regularly check your child's response to the treatment.

You have many options for treating your child's ASD. However, not all of them have been proven to work through scientific studies. Read the patient information that comes with your child's medication. Some people keep these patient inserts along with their other notes for easy reference. This is most useful when dealing with several different prescription medications. You should get all the facts about possible risks and benefits and talk to more than one expert when possible before trying a new treatment on your child.

How common is ASD?

Studies measuring autism spectrum disorder (ASD) prevalence—the number of children affected by ASD over a given time period—have reported varying results, depending on when and where the studies were conducted and how the studies defined ASD.

In a 2009 government survey on ASD prevalence, the Centers for Disease Control and Prevention (CDC) found that the rate of ASD was higher than in past U.S. studies. Based on health and school records of 8-year-olds in 14 communities throughout the country, the CDC survey found that around 1 in 110 children has ASD.[41] Boys face about four to five times higher risk than girls.

Experts disagree about whether this shows a true increase in ASD prevalence. Since the earlier studies were completed, guidelines for diagnosis have changed. Also, many more parents and doctors now know about ASD, so parents are more likely to take their children to be diagnosed, and more doctors are able to properly diagnose ASD. These and other changes may help explain some differences in prevalence numbers. Even so, the CDC report confirms other recent studies showing that more children are being diagnosed with ASD than ever before. For more information, please visit the autism section of the CDC website at http://www.cdc.gov/ncbddd/autism.

What causes ASD?

Scientists don't know the exact causes of autism spectrum disorder (ASD), but research suggests that both genes and environment play important roles.

Genetic factors

In identical twins who share the exact same genetic code, if one has ASD, the other twin also has ASD in nearly 9 out of 10 cases. If one sibling has ASD, the other siblings have 35 times the normal risk of also developing the disorder. Researchers are starting to identify particular genes that may increase the risk for ASD.[42, 43]

Still, scientists have only had some success in finding exactly which genes are involved. For more information about such cases, see the section, "What are some other conditions that children with ASD may also have?" which describes Fragile X syndrome and tuberous sclerosis.

Most people who develop ASD have no reported family history of autism, suggesting that random, rare, and possibly many gene mutations are likely to affect a person's risk.[44, 45] Any change to normal genetic information is called a mutation. Mutations can be inherited, but some arise for no reason. Mutations can be helpful, harmful, or have no effect.

Having increased genetic risk does not mean a child will definitely develop ASD. Many researchers are focusing on how various genes interact with each other and environmental factors to better understand how they increase the risk of this disorder.

Environmental factors

In medicine, "environment" refers to anything outside of the body that can affect health. This includes the air we breathe, the water we drink and bathe in, the food we eat, the medicines we take, and many other things that our bodies may come in contact with. Environment also includes our surroundings in the womb, when our mother's health directly affects our growth and earliest development.

Researchers are studying many environmental factors such as family medical conditions, parental age and other demographic factors, exposure to toxins, and complications during birth or pregnancy.[29, 46–48]

As with genes, it's likely that more than one environmental factor is involved in increasing risk for ASD. And, like genes, any one of these risk factors raises the risk by only a small amount. Most people who have been exposed to environmental risk factors do not develop ASD. The National Institute of Environmental Health Sciences is also conducting research in this area. More information is available at http://www.niehs.nih.gov/health/topics/conditions/autism/index.cfm.

Scientists are studying how certain environmental factors may affect certain genes—turning them on or off, or increasing or decreasing their normal activity. This process is called epigenetics and is providing researchers with many new ways to study how disorders like ASD develop and possibly change over time.

ASD and vaccines

Health experts recommend that children receive a number of vaccines early in life to protect against dangerous, infectious diseases, such as measles. Since pediatricians in the United States started giving these vaccines during regular checkups, the number of children getting sick, becoming disabled, or dying from these diseases has dropped to almost zero.

Children in the United States receive several vaccines during their first 2 years of life, around the same age that ASD symptoms often appear or become noticeable. A minority of parents suspect that vaccines are somehow related to their child's disorder. Some may be concerned about these vaccines due to the unproven theory that ASD may be caused by thimerosal. Thimerosal is a mercury-based chemical once added to some, but not all, vaccines to help extend their shelf life. However, except for some flu vaccines, no vaccine routinely given to preschool aged children in the United States has contained thimerosal since 2001. Despite this change, the rate of children diagnosed with ASD has continued to rise.

Other parents believe their child's illness might be linked to vaccines designed to protect against more than one disease, such as the measles-mumps-rubella (MMR) vaccine, which never contained thimerosal.

Many studies have been conducted to try to determine if vaccines are a possible cause of autism. As of 2010, none of the studies has linked autism and vaccines.[49, 50]

Following extensive hearings, a special court of Federal judges ruled against several test cases that tried to prove that vaccines containing thimerosal, either by themselves or combined with the MMR vaccine, caused autism. More information about these hearings is available on the U.S. Court of Federal Claims' website at http://www.uscfc.uscourts.gov/omnibus-autism-proceeding.

The latest information about research on autism and vaccines is available from the Centers for Disease Control and Prevention at http://cdc.gov/ncbddd/autism/topics.html. This website provides information from the Federal Government and independent organizations.

What efforts are under way to improve the detection and treatment of ASD?

How can I help a child who has ASD?

What efforts are under way to improve the detection and treatment of ASD?

Many recent research studies have focused on finding the earliest signs of autism spectrum disorder (ASD). These studies aim to help doctors diagnose children at a younger age so they can get needed interventions as quickly as possible.

For example, one early sign of ASD may be increased head size or rapid head growth. Brain imaging studies have shown that abnormal brain development beginning in an infant's first months may have a role in ASD. This theory suggests that genetic defects in growth factors, which direct proper brain development, cause the brain abnormalities seen in autism. It's possible that an infant's sudden, rapid head growth may be an early warning signal, which could help in early diagnosis and treatment or possible prevention of ASD.[51]

Current studies on ASD treatment are exploring many approaches, such as:

- A computer-based training program designed to teach children with ASD how to create and respond to facial expressions appropriately[52]
- A medication that may help improve functioning in children with Fragile X syndrome[53]
- New social interventions that can be used in the classroom or other "everyday" settings
- An intervention parents can follow to reduce and prevent ASD-related disability in children at high risk for the disorder.[54]

For more information about clinical trials on ASD funded by the National Institute of Mental Health, go to http://www.nimh.nih.gov/health/trials/autism-spectrum-disorders-pervasive-developmental-disorders.shtml.

You can read about future research plans on the Interagency Autism Coordinating Committee's (IACC's) website at http://iacc.hhs.gov. The IACC is made up of representatives of Federal agencies and members of the public and coordinates efforts within the U.S. Department of Health and Human Services concerning ASD.

How can I help a child who has ASD?

After your child is diagnosed with autism spectrum disorder (ASD), you may feel unprepared or unable to provide your child with the necessary care and education. Know that there are many treatment options, social services and programs, and other resources that can help.

Some tips that can help you and your child are:

- Keep a record of conversations, meetings with health care providers and teachers, and other sources of information. This will help you remember the different treatment options and decide which would help your child most.

- Keep a record of the doctors' reports and your child's evaluation. This information may help your child qualify for special programs.

- Contact your local health department or autism advocacy groups to learn about the special programs available in your state and local community.

- Talk with your child's pediatrician, school system, or an autism support group to find an autism expert in your area who can help you develop an intervention plan and find other local resources.

Understanding teens with ASD

The teen years can be a time of stress and confusion for any growing child, including teenagers with autism spectrum disorder (ASD).

During the teenage years, adolescents become more aware of other people and their relationships with them. While most teenagers are concerned with acne, popularity, grades, and dates, teens with ASD may become painfully aware that they are different from their peers. For some, this awareness may encourage them to learn new behaviors and try to improve their social skills. For others, hurt feelings and problems connecting with others may lead to depression, anxiety, or other mental disorders. One way that some teens with ASD may express the tension and confusion that can occur during adolescence is through increased autistic or aggressive behavior. Teens with ASD will also need support to help them understand the physical changes and sexual maturation they experience during adolescence.

If your teen seems to have trouble coping, talk with his or her doctor about possible co-occurring mental disorders and what you can do. Behavioral therapies and medications often help.

Preparing for your child's transition to adulthood

The public schools' responsibility for providing services ends when a child with ASD reaches the age of 22. At that time, some families may struggle to find jobs to match their adult child's needs. If your family cannot continue caring for an adult child at home, you may need to look for other living arrangements. For more information, see the section, "Living arrangements for adults with ASD."

Long before your child finishes school, you should search for the best programs and facilities for young adults with ASD. If you know other parents of adults with ASD, ask them about the services available in your community. Local support and advocacy groups may be able to help you find programs and services that your child is eligible to receive as an adult.

Another important part of this transition is teaching youth with ASD to self-advocate. This means that they start to take on more responsibility for their education, employment, health care, and living arrangements. Adults with ASD or other disabilities must self-advocate for their rights under the Americans with Disabilities Act at work, in higher education, in the community, and elsewhere.

Living arrangements for adults with ASD

There are many options for adults living with ASD. Helping your adult child choose the right one will largely depend on what is available in your state and local community, as well as your child's skills and symptoms. Below are some examples of living arrangements you may want to consider:

- **Independent living.** Some adults with ASD are able to live on their own. Others can live in their own home or apartment if they get help dealing with major issues, such as managing personal finances, obtaining necessary health care, and interacting with government or social service agencies. Family members, professional agencies, or other types of providers can offer this assistance.

- **Living at home.** Government funds are available for families who choose to have their adult child with ASD live at home. These programs include Supplemental Security Income, Social Security Disability Insurance, and Medicaid waivers. Information about these programs and others is available from the Social Security Administration (SSA). Make an appointment with your local SSA office to find out which programs would be right for your adult child.

- **Other home alternatives.** Some families open their homes to provide long-term care to adults with disabilities who are not related to them. If the home teaches self-care and housekeeping skills and arranges leisure activities, it is called a "skill-development" home.

- **Supervised group living.** People with disabilities often live in group homes or apartments staffed by professionals who help with basic needs. These needs often include meal preparation, housekeeping, and personal care. People who are more independent may be able to live in a home or apartment where staff only visit a few times a week. Such residents generally prepare their own meals, go to work, and conduct other daily activities on their own.

- **Long-term care facilities.** This alternative is available for those with ASD who need intensive, constant supervision.

Citations

1. *American Psychiatric Association. Diagnostic and Statistical Manual of Mental Disorders, Fourth Edition – Text Revision* (DSM-IV-TR). Washington, DC: American Psychiatric Publishing, Inc., 2000.

2. Wiggins LD, Rice CE, Baio J. Developmental regression in children with an autism spectrum disorder identified by a population-based surveillance system. *Autism*, 2009 Jul;13(4):357–74.

3. Jones W, Carr K, Klin A. Absence of preferential looking to the eyes of approaching adults predicts level of social disability in 2-year-old toddlers with autism spectrum disorder. *Archives of General Psychiatry*, 2008 Aug;65(8):946–54.

4. Klin A, Lin DJ, Gorrindo P, Ramsay G, Jones W. Two-year-olds with autism orient to non-social contingencies rather than biological motion. *Nature*, 2009 May 14;459(7244):257–61.

5. Ben Zeev Ghidoni B. Rett syndrome. *Child and Adolescent Psychiatric Clinics of North America*, 2007 Jul;16(3):723–43.

6. Percy AK. Rett syndrome. Current status and new vistas. *Neurologic Clinics*, 2002 Nov;20(4):1125–41.

7. Fombonne E. Prevalence of childhood disintegrative disorder. *Autism*, 2002 Jun;6(2):149–57.

8. *Eunice Kennedy Shriver* National Institute of Child Health and Human Development, NIH, DHHS. *Rett Syndrome*. Washington, DC: U.S. Government Printing Office, NIH-06-5590, 2006.

9. Fombonne E. Epidemiology of autistic disorder and other pervasive developmental disorders. *Journal of Clinical Psychiatry*, 2005; 66(Suppl 10):3–8.

10. Volkmar FR, Rutter M. Childhood disintegrative disorder: results of the DSM-IV autism field trial. Journal of the *American Academy of Child and Adolescent Psychiatry*, 1995 Aug;34(8):1092–5.

11. Volkmar FR. "Childhood Disintegrative Disorder - Case Report." in Spitzer RL. (ed) *DSM-IV Casebook*. Washington, DC: American Psychiatric Press, 1994.

12. Filipek PA, Accardo PJ, Ashwal S, Baranek GT, Cook EH, Jr., Dawson G, Gordon B, Gravel JS, Johnson CP, Kallen RJ, Levy SE, Minshew NJ, Ozonoff S, Prizant BM, Rapin I, Rogers SJ, Stone WL, Teplin SW, Tuchman RF, Volkmar FR. Practice parameter: screening and diagnosis of autism: report of the Quality Standards Subcommittee of the American Academy of Neurology and the Child Neurology Society. *Neurology*, 2000 Aug 22;55(4):468–79.

13. Landa RJ, Holman KC, Garrett-Mayer E. Social and communication development in toddlers with early and later diagnosis of autism spectrum disorders. *Archives of General Psychiatry*, 2007 Jul;64(7):853–64.

14. Johnson CP, Myers SM. Identification and evaluation of children with autism spectrum disorders. *Pediatrics*, 2007 Nov;120(5):1183–215.

15. Krakowiak P, Goodlin-Jones B, Hertz-Picciotto I, Croen LA, Hansen RL. Sleep problems in children with autism spectrum disorders, developmental delays, and typical development: a population-based study. *Journal of Sleep Research*, 2008 Jun;17(2):197–206.

16. Johnson KP, Giannotti F, Cortesi F. Sleep patterns in autism spectrum disorders. *Child and Adolescent Psychiatric Clinics of North America*, 2009 Oct;18(4):917–28.

17. Volkmar FR. "Medical Problems, Treatments, and Professionals." in Powers MD. (ed) *Children with Autism: A Parent's Guide, Second Edition*. Bethesda: Woodbine House, 2000.

18. Zafeiriou DI, Ververi A, Vargiami E. Childhood autism and associated comorbidities. *Brain and Development*, 2007 Jun;29(5):257–72.

19. *Eunice Kennedy Shriver* National Institute of Child Health and Human Development, NIH, PHS, DHHS *Families and Fragile X Syndrome*. Washington, DC: U.S. Government Printing Office, NIH-96-3402, 2003.

20. Smalley SL. Autism and tuberous sclerosis. *Journal of Autism and Developmental Disorders*, 1998 Oct;28(5):407–14.

21. Xue M, Brimacombe M, Chaaban J, Zimmerman-Bier B, Wagner GC. Autism spectrum disorders: concurrent clinical disorders. *Journal of Child Neurology*, 2008 Jan;23(1):6–13.

22. Kuddo T, Nelson KB. How common are gastrointestinal disorders in children with autism? *Current Opinion in Pediatrics*, 2003 Jun;15(3):339–43.

23. Nikolov RN, Bearss KE, Lettinga J, Erickson C, Rodowski M, Aman MG, McCracken JT, McDougle CJ, Tierney E, Vitiello B, Arnold LE, Shah B, Posey DJ, Ritz L, Scahill L. Gastrointestinal symptoms in a sample of children with pervasive developmental disorders. *Journal of Autism and Developmental Disorders*, 2009 Mar;39(3):405–13.

24. Buie T, Campbell DB, Fuchs GJ, 3rd, Furuta GT, Levy J, Vandewater J, Whitaker AH, Atkins D, Bauman ML, Beaudet AL, Carr EG, Gershon MD, Hyman SL, Jirapinyo P, Jyonouchi H, Kooros K, Kushak R, Levitt P, Levy SE, Lewis JD, Murray KF, Natowicz MR, Sabra A, Wershil BK, Weston SC, Zeltzer L, Winter H. Evaluation, diagnosis, and treatment of gastrointestinal disorders in individuals with ASDs: a consensus report. *Pediatrics*, 2010 Jan;125 Suppl 1:S1–18.

25. Leyfer OT, Folstein SE, Bacalman S, Davis NO, Dinh E, Morgan J, Tager-Flusberg H, Lainhart JE. Comorbid psychiatric disorders in children with autism: interview development and rates of disorders. *Journal of Autism and Developmental Disorders*, 2006 Oct;36(7):849–61.

26. Simonoff E, Pickles A, Charman T, Chandler S, Loucas T, Baird G. Psychiatric disorders in children with autism spectrum disorders: prevalence, comorbidity, and associated factors in a population-derived sample. *Journal of the American Academy of Child and Adolescent Psychiatry*, 2008 Aug;47(8):921–9.

27. Reichow B, Wolery M. Comprehensive synthesis of early intensive behavioral interventions for young children with autism based on the UCLA young autism project model. *Journal of Autism and Developmental Disorders*, 2009 Jan;39(1):23–41.

28. Rogers SJ, Vismara LA. Evidence-based comprehensive treatments for early autism. *Journal of Clinical Child and Adolescent Psychology*, 2008 Jan;37(1):8–38.

29. Myers SM, Johnson CP. Management of children with autism spectrum disorders. *Pediatrics*, 2007 Nov;120(5):1162–82.

30. McEachin JJ, Smith T, Lovaas OI. Long-term outcome for children with autism who received early intensive behavioral treatment. *American Journal of Mental Retardation*, 1993 Jan;97(4):359-72; discussion 73–91.

31. Couper JJ, Sampson AJ. Children with autism deserve evidence-based intervention. *Medical Journal of Australia*, 2003 May 5;178(9):424–5.

32. Levy SE, Mandell DS, Schultz RT. Autism. *Lancet*, 2009 Nov 7;374(9701):1627–38.

33. Paul R. Interventions to improve communication in autism. *Child and Adolescent Psychiatric Clinics of North America*, 2008 Oct;17(4):835-56, ix–x.

34. Autism Speaks. How Is Autism Treated? http://www. autismspeaks.org/docs/family_services_docs/100day2/ Treatment_Version_2_0.pdf. Accessed on October 22, 2010.

35. The Interdisciplinary Council on Developmental and Learning Disorders. Floortime overview. http://www.icdl.com/ dirFloortime/overview/index.shtml. Accessed on Jun 17, 2009.

36. TEACCH – UNC School of Medicine. What is TEACCH? http:// teacch.com/about-us-1/what-is-teacch. Accessed on Jun 17, 2009.

37. Bellini S, Peters JK. Social skills training for youth with autism spectrum disorders. *Child and Adolescent Psychiatric Clinics of North America*, 2008 Oct;17(4):857–73.

38. Frankel F, Myatt R, Sugar C, Whitham C, Gorospe CM, Laugeson E. A Randomized Controlled Study of Parent-assisted Children's Friendship Training with Children having Autism Spectrum Disorders. *Journal of Autism and Developmental Disorders*, 2010 Jul;40(7):827–42.

39. King BH, Hollander E, Sikich L, McCracken JT, Scahill L, Bregman JD, Donnelly CL, Anagnostou E, Dukes K, Sullivan L, Hirtz D, Wagner A, Ritz L. Lack of efficacy of citalopram in children with autism spectrum disorders and high levels of repetitive behavior: citalopram ineffective in children with autism. *Archives of General Psychiatry*, 2009 Jun;66(6): 583–90.

40. Research Units on Pediatric Psychopharmacology Autism Network. Randomized, controlled, crossover trial of methylphenidate in pervasive developmental disorders with hyperactivity. *Archives of General Psychiatry*, 2005 Nov;62(11):1266–74.

41. Prevalence of autism spectrum disorders - Autism and Developmental Disabilities Monitoring Network, United States, 2006. *MMWR Surveillance Summaries*, 2009 Dec 18;58(10):1–20.

42. Campbell DB, Sutcliffe JS, Ebert PJ, Militerni R, Bravaccio C, Trillo S, Elia M, Schneider C, Melmed R, Sacco R, Persico AM, Levitt P. A genetic variant that disrupts MET transcription is associated with autism. *Proceedings of the National Academy of Sciences of the United States of America*, 2006 Nov 7;103(45):16834–9.

43. Arking DE, Cutler DJ, Brune CW, Teslovich TM, West K, Ikeda M, Rea A, Guy M, Lin S, Cook EH, Chakravarti A. A common genetic variant in the neurexin superfamily member CNTNAP2 increases familial risk of autism. *American Journal of Human Genetics*, 2008 Jan;82(1):160–4.

44. Sebat J, Lakshmi B, Malhotra D, Troge J, Lese-Martin C, Walsh T, Yamrom B, Yoon S, Krasnitz A, Kendall J, Leotta A, Pai D, Zhang R, Lee YH, Hicks J, Spence SJ, Lee AT, Puura K, Lehtimaki T, Ledbetter D, Gregersen PK, Bregman J, Sutcliffe JS, Jobanputra V, Chung W, Warburton D, King MC, Skuse D, Geschwind DH, Gilliam TC, Ye K, Wigler M. Strong association of de novo copy number mutations with autism. *Science*, 2007 Apr 20;316(5823):445–9.

45. Morrow EM, Yoo SY, Flavell SW, Kim TK, Lin Y, Hill RS, Mukaddes NM, Balkhy S, Gascon G, Hashmi A, Al-Saad S, Ware J, Joseph RM, Greenblatt R, Gleason D, Ertelt JA, Apse KA, Bodell A, Partlow JN, Barry B, Yao H, Markianos K, Ferland RJ, Greenberg ME, Walsh CA. Identifying autism loci and genes by tracing recent shared ancestry. *Science*, 2008 Jul 11;321(5886):218–23.

46. Kolevzon A, Gross R, Reichenberg A. Prenatal and perinatal risk factors for autism: a review and integration of findings. *Archives of Pediatric and Adolescent Medicine*, 2007 Apr;161(4):326–33.

47. Lawler CP, Croen LA, Grether JK, Van de Water J. Identifying environmental contributions to autism: provocative clues and false leads. *Mental Retardation and Developmental Disabilities Research Reviews*, 2004;10(4):292–302.

48. Daniels JL, Forssen U, Hultman CM, Cnattingius S, Savitz DA, Feychting M, Sparen P. Parental psychiatric disorders associated with autism spectrum disorders in the offspring. *Pediatrics*, 2008 May;121(5):e1357–62.

49. Immunization Safety Review Committee. *Immunization Safety Review: Vaccines and Autism*. Washington, DC: The National Academies Press; 2004.

50. Interagency Autism Coordinating Committee. Question 3: what caused this to happen and can this be prevented? *The 2010 Interagency Autism Coordinating Committee Strategic Plan for Autism Spectrum Disorders Research – January, 19, 2010*. Washington, DC: Interagency Autism Coordinating Committee, U.S. Department of Health and Human Services, 2010.

51. Courchesne E, Carper R, Akshoomoff N. Evidence of brain overgrowth in the first year of life in autism. *JAMA*. 2003 Jul 16;290(3):337–44.

52. National Institute of Mental Health. Recovery act grant aims to teach kids with autism how to better express themselves. http://www.nimh.nih.gov/science-news/2009/recovery-act-grant-aims-to-teach-kids-with-autism-how-to-better-express-themselves.shtml. Accessed on March 23, 2010.

53. National Institute of Mental Health. Clinical tests begin on medication to correct Fragile X defect. http://www.nimh.nih. gov/science-news/2009/clinical-tests-begin-on-medication-to-correct-fragile-x-defect.shtml. Accessed on March 23, 2010.

54. National Institute of Mental Health. NIH awards more than 50 grants to boost search for causes, improve treatments for autism. http://www.nimh.nih.gov/science-news/2009/ nih-awards-more-than-50-grants-to-boost-search-for-causes-improve-treatments-for-autism.shtml. Accessed on March 23, 2010.

This guide is intended to help parents understand what autism spectrum disorder (ASD) is, recognize common signs and symptoms, and find the resources they need. It's important to remember that help is available.

Reprints

This publication is in the public domain and may be reproduced or copied without permission from NIMH. We encourage you to reproduce it and use it in your efforts to improve public health. Citation of the National Institute of Mental Health as a source is appreciated. However, using government materials inappropriately can raise legal or ethical concerns, so we ask you to use these guidelines:

- NIMH does not endorse or recommend any commercial products, processes, or services, and our publications may not be used for advertising or endorsement purposes.

- NIMH does not provide specific medical advice or treatment recommendations or referrals; our materials may not be used in a manner that has the appearance of such information.

- NIMH requests that non-Federal organizations not alter our publications in ways that will jeopardize the integrity and "brand" when using the publication.

- Addition of non-Federal Government logos and website links may not have the appearance of NIMH endorsement of any specific commercial products or services or medical treatments or services.

If you have questions regarding these guidelines and use of NIMH publications, please contact the NIMH Information Resource Center at 1-866-615-6464 or e-mail at nimhinfo@nih.gov.

For More Information on Autism Spectrum Disorder

Visit the National Library of Medicine's MedlinePlus
http://medlineplus.gov

En Español
http://medlineplus.gov/spanish

For information on clinical trials
http://www.nimh.nih.gov/health/trials/index.shtml

National Library of Medicine clinical trials database
http://www.clinicaltrials.gov

Information from NIMH is available in multiple formats.
You can browse online, download documents in PDF,
and order materials through the mail. Check the NIMH
Website at **http://www.nimh.nih.gov** for the latest
information on this topic and to order publications.
If you do not have Internet access please contact the
NIMH Information Resource Center at the numbers listed
below.

National Institute of Mental Health
Science Writing, Press & Dissemination Branch
6001 Executive Boulevard
Room 8184, MSC 9663
Bethesda, MD 20892-9663
Phone: 301-443-4513 or
    1-866-615-NIMH (6464) toll-free
TTY: 301-443-8431 or
    866-415-8051 toll-free
FAX: 301-443-4279
E-mail: **nimhinfo@nih.gov**
Website: **http://www.nimh.nih.gov**

23930876R00016

Made in the USA
Lexington, KY
04 July 2013